PREGNANCY RED FLAGS

A Comprehensive Guide to Recognizing

and Responding to Warning Signs

During Pregnancy

Cheryl Everett

Table of Content

INTRODUCTION

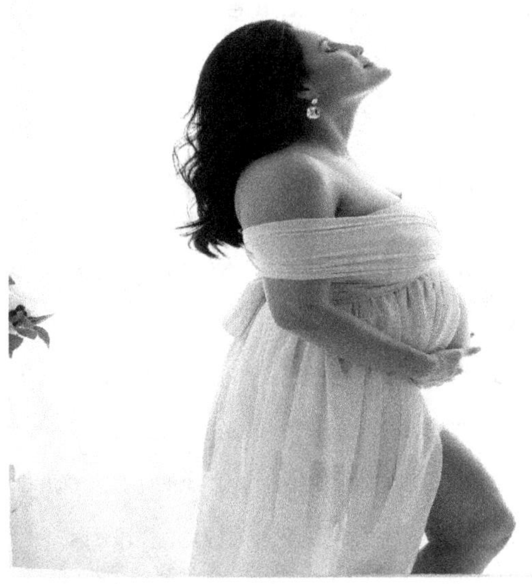

Pregnancy is a remarkable and transformative experience in a woman's life, characterized by the gradual development of a new human being within her body. While it is typically a time of great anticipation and joy, it is also marked by numerous physical, emotional, and physiological changes, making it essential for expectant mothers, their partners, and healthcare providers to be vigilant for potential red flags that could signal complications or health concerns. These "pregnancy red flags" refer to signs and symptoms that may indicate underlying issues and require immediate attention to safeguard the well-being of both the mother and the developing fetus.

Recognizing these red flags is crucial because pregnancy is not without its risks. Even though modern medical care has significantly improved maternal and fetal outcomes, complications can still arise, some of which may be life-threatening if left unaddressed. These red flags may vary in severity and can encompass a wide range of conditions, from common discomforts and minor concerns to more serious issues, including but not limited to preeclampsia, gestational diabetes, placental abnormalities, preterm labor, and fetal distress.

In this guide, we will explore 15 various aspects of pregnancy red flags, from common indicators such as morning sickness and swelling to more critical conditions like bleeding during pregnancy or decreased fetal movement. We will delve into the importance of regular prenatal care, which plays a central role in the early detection and management of potential red flags, as well as the essential role of healthcare providers and expectant mothers in monitoring and responding to these warning signs.

Furthermore, we will emphasize the significance of individualized care during pregnancy, as every woman's experience is unique. While certain red flags may be common, their severity and impact can vary from person to person. This highlights the need for open communication between pregnant individuals and their healthcare teams, fostering an environment of trust and shared decision-making to address these concerns effectively.

This discussion aims to provide a comprehensive overview of pregnancy red flags, the reasons for vigilance during this extraordinary journey, and the measures to take to ensure the safety and well-being of both mother and child. By being informed and proactive, expectant mothers and their healthcare providers can work together to minimize risks and complications, ultimately leading to a healthier and more positive pregnancy experience.

This guide is a reminder that being vigilant during pregnancy is not a cause for panic, but an act of love and care for both Mother and baby

CHAPTER ONE

Stages in Pregnancies

Pregnancy unfolds in distinct stages, each marked by unique developments and milestones. These stages are crucial for both the mother's and baby's well-being.Pregnancy typically consists of three main stages, known as trimesters, each with its own set of changes and developments. Here's a comprehensive overview of each stage and what to expect:

First Trimester (Week 1 to Week 12):

1. Conception: Pregnancy begins with conception when a sperm fertilizes an egg, forming a zygote.This typically occurs when a woman's ovary releases an egg (ovulation) and it meets a sperm in the fallopian tube.
2. Implantation: The fertilized egg implants into the uterine wall, and the placenta starts to form.

3. Symptoms: Early pregnancy symptoms may include fatigue, breast tenderness, nausea (morning sickness), frequent urination, and mood swings.
4. Development: Organs and major body systems start to form. The heartbeat becomes detectable, and the embryo is now referred to as a fetus.
5. Medical Care: Women typically start prenatal care during this stage, which includes regular check-ups, ultrasounds, and blood tests.

The first prenatal appointments and ultrasounds take place, confirming the pregnancy and estimating the due date.

Second Trimester (Week 13 to Week 28):

1. Growth and Movement: The fetus begins to grow rapidly, and the mother usually starts feeling fetal movements, commonly known

as "quickening."The baby continues to grow, and the mother's belly begins to visibly show the pregnancy

2. Symptoms: Morning sickness often improves, but new symptoms may arise, such as backaches, leg cramps, and skin changes.
3. Ultrasound: A detailed ultrasound can reveal the baby's sex and check for any developmental abnormalities.
4. Viability: The fetus becomes viable (able to survive outside the womb) around the 24th week.
5. Medical Care: Regular check-ups continue, and screening tests for genetic disorders may be offered.

Third Trimester (Week 29 to Birth):

1. Rapid Growth: The fetus continues to grow, and the mother's body undergoes significant changes to prepare for childbirth.The baby's

rapid growth continues, and major organs like the brain and lungs mature.

2. Symptoms: Swelling, discomfort , difficulty sleeping, shortness of breath, heartburn, and frequent urination become more pronounced. Braxton Hicks contractions may occur.

3. The mother may experience discomfort, including backaches, swelling, and difficulty sleeping

4. Preparation for Birth: The baby typically settles into a head-down position in the pelvis. Preparation for Birth: The baby typically settles into a head-down position in the pelvis. The cervix begins to abolish and dilate.

5. Medical Care: More frequent check-ups are scheduled. Birth plans and preferences are discussed.

6. Labor and Birth: Contractions, which become regular and more painful, signal the onset of labor. Labor involves uterine contractions that help the baby move through the birth canal.

7. Stages of labor include dilation and effacement of the cervix, the birth of the baby, and the delivery of the placenta.
8. This culminates in the miraculous moment when the baby takes its first breath outside the womb

Each stage of pregnancy is a unique and vital part of the journey, marked by specific changes and milestones. It's crucial for expectant mothers to receive prenatal care and support throughout these stages to ensure a healthy and safe pregnancy for both the mother and the baby. These stages provide a framework for understanding the journey of pregnancy. Each trimester brings its unique joys and challenges, ultimately leading to the miraculous moment of childbirth. It's important for expectant mothers to receive regular prenatal care and support from healthcare providers throughout these stages to ensure a healthy and safe pregnancy.

CHAPTER TWO

Pregnancy Red Flags: Identifying Warning signs in Pregnancies

Pregnancy is a remarkable journey, but it can also come with potential complications that require vigilant attention. Identifying warning signs in pregnancy is crucial for the well-being of both the expectant mother and her baby. In this comprehensive guide, we will explore the critical warning signs that every pregnant woman, her family, and healthcare providers should be aware of. Pregnancy red flags are critical signs and symptoms that expectant mothers should be aware of during their pregnancy. These indicators may suggest potential complications and should prompt immediate medical attention. It's important to remember that every pregnancy is unique, and what constitutes a red flag can vary from person to person. Nevertheless, here are some common pregnancy warning signs.

1. VAGINA BLEEDING

Any quantity of vaginal bleeding during pregnancy should be taken very seriously. While some light spotting can be normal, heavy bleeding may indicate issues such as a miscarriage, ectopic pregnancy, or placental problems.

Types of Vaginal Bleeding:

- Implantation Bleeding: This is a light spotting that can occur when the fertilized egg attaches to the uterine lining, typically around 6-12 days after conception.
- Spotting: Light bleeding or spotting can happen at any point during pregnancy. It might be due to cervical changes, irritation, or other benign factors.
- First Trimester Bleeding: Bleeding in the first trimester is more common and can be caused by various factors, including miscarriage,

ectopic pregnancy, or molar
pregnancy.

Ectopic Pregnancy :This is a
pregnancy in which the fertilized egg
implants outside the uterus.

Molar Pregnancy: this occurs when
placental tissue swells and appear to
form fluid filled cysts.

- Second and Third Trimester
  Bleeding: Bleeding in the later
  stages of pregnancy may be due to
  issues like placenta previa, placental
  abruption, or preterm labor.

Causes of Vaginal Bleeding in Pregnancy:

- Miscarriage: Heavy bleeding, along
  with cramping and abdominal pain,
  can indicate a miscarriage.

- Ectopic Pregnancy: When a fertilized egg implants outside the uterus, it can cause bleeding and severe abdominal pain.
- Placental Issues: Placenta previa (low-lying placenta) and placental abruption (separation of the placenta from the uterine wall) can lead to bleeding.
- Cervical Changes: Hormonal changes and increased blood flow can cause the cervix to be more sensitive and prone to bleeding.
- Infections or Conditions: Infections of the cervix or vagina, such as yeast infections, can cause bleeding. Conditions like cervical polyps or fibroids may also lead to bleeding.

Management of Vagina Bleeding in pregnancy

When to Seek Medical Help:

- Any Amount of vaginal bleeding during pregnancy must be reported to a healthcare provider for proper check up.
- Heavy bleeding (soaking through a pad in an hour or less) or bleeding associated with severe pain should be addressed immediately.
- Seek prompt medical attention if you experience dizziness, fainting, or signs of shock along with bleeding.

Diagnosis and Treatment:

- A healthcare provider will perform a physical exam, and possibly an

ultrasound, to determine the cause
of the bleeding.

- o   Treatment depends on the
  underlying cause. Some conditions,
  like cervical bleeding or minor
  placental issues, may resolve on
  their own. In more serious cases,
  medical or surgical intervention may
  be necessary.

Preventing Vaginal Bleeding:

- o   Attend regular prenatal check-ups to
  monitor the health of both you and
  the baby.
- o   Follow your doctor's advice
  regarding lifestyle and activity
  restrictions, especially if you have a
  high-risk pregnancy.

Vaginal bleeding during pregnancy is a concerning symptom that should never be ignored. It can be an indication of both benign and serious conditions, and it's essential to seek prompt medical evaluation to ensure the health and well-being of both the mother and the baby. Your healthcare provider can provide the most accurate diagnosis and treatment plan based on the specific circumstances of your pregnancy.

2. SEVERE ABDOMINAL PAIN

Severe abdominal pain during pregnancy can be a cause for concern, as it may indicate various underlying issues. It's essential to promptly consult with a healthcare provider when experiencing severe abdominal pain while pregnant, as it could signal a potentially serious condition. Here are some common **causes of severe abdominal pain during pregnancy**:

1. Ectopic gravidity: An ectopic gravidity occurs when the fertilized egg implants outside the uterus, generally in the fallopian tube. This can cause severe abdominal pain, often on one side, and is a medical emergency.
2. Miscarriage: Severe abdominal pain accompanied by bleeding can be a sign of a

miscarriage, which is the loss of the pregnancy before the 20th week. It is necessary to seek immediate medical attention in this situation.

3. Round Ligament Pain: This is a common cause of abdominal discomfort during pregnancy. The round ligaments that support the uterus can stretch and cause sharp, stabbing pains, especially when changing position or with sudden movements.

4. Gastrointestinal Issues: Constipation, gas, or indigestion can lead to significant discomfort, often mistaken for abdominal pain. Hormonal changes in pregnancy can slow down digestion, exacerbating these issues.

5. Braxton Hicks Contractions: These are often referred to as "false labor" contractions and can cause abdominal discomfort. They are usually irregular and less painful than true labor contractions.

6. Placental Abruption: In this serious condition, the placenta partially or

completely detaches from the uterus before childbirth. Severe abdominal pain, often accompanied by bleeding, is a hallmark symptom.

7. Urinary Tract Infections (UTIs): UTIs can cause lower abdominal pain and discomfort. They should be treated promptly as untreated UTIs can lead to more severe issues.

8. Preeclampsia: Preeclampsia is a potentially serious pregnancy complication characterized by high blood pressure and damage to organs, often the liver and kidneys. It can cause abdominal pain, typically in the upper right side, along with other symptoms like swelling and headaches.

Management of severe Abdominal pain

It's crucial to differentiate between normal pregnancy discomfort and severe abdominal pain. Any severe or persistent abdominal pain should be evaluated by a healthcare provider. They will perform a thorough examination, which may include ultrasounds, blood tests, and other diagnostic procedures to determine the cause and develop an appropriate treatment plan.

In many cases, early detection and treatment can mitigate potential complications. Pregnant individuals should always maintain open communication with their healthcare provider and seek medical attention promptly if they experience severe abdominal pain or any other concerning symptoms during pregnancy.

3. SEVERE HEADACHE AND HIGH FEVER

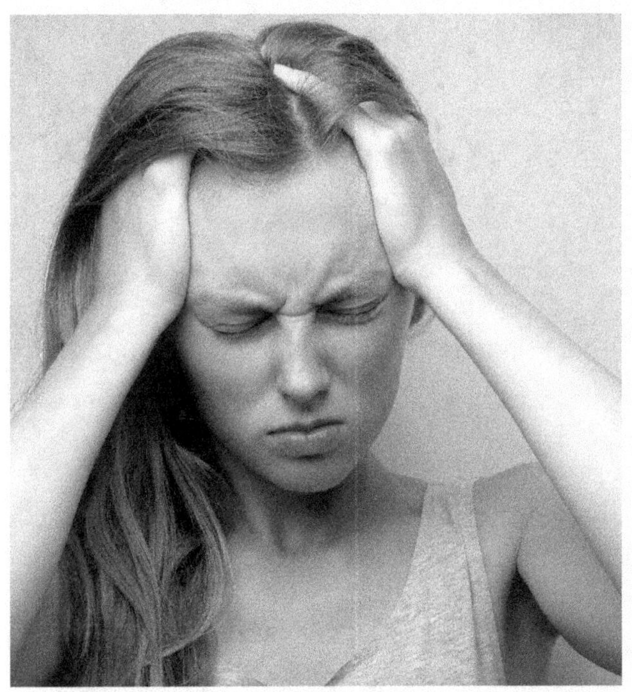

Severe Headaches in pregnancy

- Causes: Severe headaches during
  pregnancy can have various causes,
  including hormonal changes, increased

blood volume, sinus congestion, tension, and even migraines. In some cases, severe headaches can be a sign of more serious conditions.

- Warning Signs: While headaches are common in pregnancy, severe and persistent headaches can be a red flag. They could be a symptom of conditions such as preeclampsia or eclampsia, which are characterized by high blood pressure and can be life-threatening if not managed.

- Treatment: The treatment for severe headaches in pregnancy depends on the underlying cause. In many cases, simple remedies like rest, hydration, relaxation techniques, and pain relief medication (as recommended by a healthcare professional) can help. However, for more serious conditions like preeclampsia, prompt medical intervention is required.

High Fever in Pregnancy:

- Causes: Fever during pregnancy can result from infections, such as the flu, urinary tract infections, or other illnesses. Infections that cause fever should be treated promptly, as they can have adverse effects on both the mother and the baby.
- pitfalls/Risks: High fever during gestation, especially during the first trimester, can increase the threat of birth blights.. It's essential to control fever to minimize potential harm to the developing fetus.
- Treatment: If you have a high fever during pregnancy, it's crucial to contact your healthcare provider immediately. They will help determine the cause of the fever and recommend appropriate treatment, which may involve antibiotics or antiviral medications, depending on the underlying condition.

Experiencing severe headaches and high fever during pregnancy can be concerning, and it's essential to consult with a healthcare professional. They can assess the situation, conduct necessary tests, and provide guidance on how to manage and treat these symptoms. Early intervention is crucial to ensure the health and well-being of both the mother and the unborn child.

4. REDUCED FETAL MOVEMENT

Reduced fetal movement in pregnancy, often referred to as decreased fetal movement (DFM), is a concern that many expectant mothers may experience. It can be a source of anxiety, but it's essential to understand the causes, potential risks, and when to seek medical attention.

Causes of Reduced Fetal Movement:

1. Normal Variations: It's important to note that there are natural variations in fetal movement. The frequency and intensity of fetal movements can vary from one pregnancy to another and may depend on factors like the position of the baby, the mother's activity level, and the gestational age.
2. Sleep Cycles: Babies in the womb have sleep-wake cycles, and they may have quieter periods when they are resting. It's

common for babies to have periods of
reduced movement during these times.

3. Maternal Factors: Factors such as the
mother's body mass index (BMI), the
location of the placenta, and the amount of
amniotic fluid can influence how movements
are felt. For example, a mother with more
abdominal fat may feel movements later in
pregnancy.

Risks and Concerns:

While reduced fetal movement can be entirely
normal, it can also be a sign of potential issues,
and therefore, it's crucial to be vigilant and consult
a healthcare provider when you notice a significant
decrease in movement. Here are some reasons for
concern:

1. Fetal Distress: Reduced movement may
indicate fetal distress. The baby may not be
getting enough oxygen or nutrients, possibly

due to a problem with the placenta or umbilical cord.

2. Positional Issues: The baby's position in the womb can sometimes limit their ability to move. This can be addressed through medical intervention or repositioning techniques.

3. Growth Restriction: In some cases, DFM can be a sign of intrauterine growth restriction (IUGR), where the baby isn't growing at the expected rate. This may be due to various factors, including placental problems or genetic issues.

4. Infection or Illness: In rare cases, infections or illnesses in the mother can lead to reduced fetal movement.

When to Seek Medical Attention:

Expectant mothers should be aware of the importance of monitoring their baby's movements and contact their healthcare provider if they notice a significant reduction.

Guidelines for when to seek medical attention
include:

1. If you notice a significant drop in fetal
    movement
2. If you feel no movement for an extended
    period, typically after 24 weeks of
    pregnancy.
3. If you're concerned about changes in the
    pattern of movements, such as a decrease
    in frequency, intensity, or a change from
    regular to irregular movements.

Medical Evaluation:

When you contact your healthcare provider due to
reduced fetal movement, they will likely perform
various assessments, which may include:

1. Fetal Monitoring: This can involve using a
    handheld Doppler device, electronic fetal

monitoring (EFM), or ultrasound to check the baby's heart rate and movements.

2. Non-Stress Test (NST): NST is a common test to assess fetal well-being. It monitors the baby's heart rate in response to their movements.

3. Biophysical Profile (BPP): A BPP combines ultrasound and NST to provide a more comprehensive evaluation of the baby's well-being.

4. Amniotic Fluid Assessment: An ultrasound may be used to assess the level of amniotic fluid, as reduced fluid can impact fetal movements.

5. Additional Tests: Depending on the circumstances, further tests may be conducted to identify the cause of DFM.

Reduced fetal movement in pregnancy is a significant concern, but it's not always a cause for alarm. Most of the time, it's due to natural variations, but it's crucial to consult a healthcare provider timely to rule out any potential problems.

5. SWELLING AND EDEMA

Swelling and edema are common symptoms experienced by many pregnant women. These conditions occur due to various physiological changes that take place during pregnancy, including increased blood volume, hormonal fluctuations, and the pressure exerted by the growing uterus on blood vessels. Let's delve into these topics more extensively:

1.Understanding Edema:

- Definition: Edema refers to the excessive accumulation of fluid in the body's tissues, leading to swelling. In pregnancy, it often occurs in the lower extremities, such as the ankles, feet, and sometimes the hands.

2. Causes of Edema in Pregnancy:

  - Hormonal Changes: The body produces more hormones, like progesterone, which can lead to increased fluid retention.

- o Blood Volume Expansion: During pregnancy, the body produces more blood to support the growing fetus, which can lead to fluid accumulation.
- o Uterine Pressure: The growing uterus can exert pressure on the pelvic blood vessels, restricting blood flow from the legs back to the heart. This can contribute to edema in the lower limbs.
- o graveness: Fluid tends to accumulate in the lower extremities due to the impact of gravity

3. Managing Edema in Pregnancy:
- o Stay Hydrated: Drinking plenty of water can help flush excess sodium and waste from the body, reducing edema.
- o Elevate Legs: Elevating the legs when possible can help reduce swelling.
- o Compression Stockings: Wearing compression stockings can provide

support to the blood vessels and
reduce fluid accumulation.

- Regular Exercise: Gentle,
  low-impact exercise can improve
  circulation and reduce edema.
- Reduce Sodium Intake: Excess
  sodium can lead to fluid retention, so
  it's important to monitor sodium
  consumption.
- Prenatal Care: Regular prenatal
  check-ups allow healthcare
  providers to monitor and address
  edema if it becomes severe.

4. When to Seek Medical Attention:

- While mild edema is common during
  pregnancy, severe swelling,
  particularly in the face and hands,
  could be a sign of preeclampsia, a
  serious pregnancy-related condition.
  If you experience rapid and severe
  swelling, high blood pressure, or
  other concerning symptoms, it's
  important to contact your healthcare
  provider immediately.

5. Swelling in Different Trimesters:

- Swelling and edema can vary in intensity throughout the pregnancy. It's often more pronounced in the third trimester due to the increased pressure on blood vessels and the significant expansion of blood volume.

6. Postpartum Edema:

- Some degree of swelling can persist after childbirth. It's important to continue hydrating and elevating your legs to help reduce postpartum edema.

Swelling and edema are common discomforts during pregnancy, primarily due to hormonal changes, increased blood volume, and uterine pressure on blood vessels. While mild edema is typical, it's crucial to monitor and manage it, and contact your healthcare provider if you experience severe or sudden swelling to rule out any underlying complications.

6. PERSISTENT NAUSEA AND VOMITING

Persistent nausea and vomiting during pregnancy, commonly referred to as morning sickness, can be a challenging and uncomfortable condition that affects many pregnant women. While it's often called "morning sickness," it can actually occur at any time of the day or night and vary in severity from woman to woman. In more severe cases, it is diagnosed as hyperemesis gravidarum, a condition that requires medical attention. Here is an extensive discussion of persistent nausea and vomiting in pregnancy:

Prevalence and Timing:

1.Morning sickness is a common symptom of early pregnancy and typically begins around the 6th week, peaking around the 9th to 13th weeks, and gradually subsiding by the second trimester. still, some women may witness it throughout their entire gestation

Symptoms:

Morning sickness is characterized by nausea, vomiting, and an aversion to certain foods and smells. The severity of these symptoms can vary widely, from mild queasiness to severe, frequent vomiting.

Causes:

Morning sickness can likely occur as a result of combination of hormonal changes, particularly increased levels of human chorionic gonadotropin (hCG) and estrogen, as well as psychological and genetic factors.

Risk Factors:

Some factors can increase the likelihood of experiencing severe morning sickness, such as a history of motion sickness, multiple pregnancies (e.g., twins or triplets), and a family history of nausea during pregnancy.

Impact on Pregnancy:

While morning sickness is generally not harmful to the fetus, severe and persistent vomiting can lead to dehydration, electrolyte imbalances, and weight loss, which can affect both the mother and the developing baby. In such cases, it's essential to seek medical care.

Management and Treatment:

1. Managing morning sickness involves a combination of lifestyle changes and

medical interventions. Recommendations include eating small, frequent meals, staying hydrated, getting plenty of rest, and avoiding triggers that worsen symptoms.

2. Medications: In cases of severe morning sickness or hyperemesis gravidarum, healthcare providers may prescribe antiemetic medications to help control nausea and vomiting. These are advised to be used under medical supervision.

3. Alternative Therapies: Some women find relief through alternative therapies like acupuncture, acupressure, ginger supplements, or wristbands designed to alleviate nausea.

4. Nutritional Supplements: Prenatal vitamins and supplements containing vitamin B6 and ginger may help alleviate symptoms.

5. When to Seek Medical Help: Persistent nausea and vomiting should be discussed with a healthcare provider. If it leads to dehydration, significant weight loss, or interferes with daily life, immediate medical attention is necessary.

6. Psychological Impact: The emotional and psychological toll of persistent morning sickness should not be underestimated. It can lead to stress, anxiety, and indeed depression. Support from healthcare professionals, family, and musketeers is pivotal.

7. Postpartum Resolution: Morning sickness usually resolves after childbirth. For some women, it disappears immediately, while others may experience it for a short period postpartum.

While morning sickness is a common and often temporary discomfort during pregnancy, persistent nausea and vomiting, particularly when severe, should be taken seriously and managed under the guidance of a healthcare provider. Seeking medical attention early can prevent complications and ensure a healthier pregnancy for both the mother and the baby.

7. PRETERM LABOR

Preterm labor, also known as premature labor, is a critical issue in pregnancy. It occurs when a woman goes into labor and begins dilating before reaching 37 weeks of gestation. Full-term pregnancy typically lasts around 40 weeks, and babies born before 37 weeks are considered premature. Preterm birth can pose significant health risks to the baby and is a leading cause of neonatal mortality and long-term health problems. Understanding the causes, risk factors, symptoms, and management of preterm labor is essential for expectant mothers and healthcare providers.

Causes of Preterm Labor:

1. Infection: Infections in the genital or urinary tract can trigger an inflammatory response that may lead to preterm contractions.

2. Multiple Pregnancies: Women carrying twins or higher-order multiples are at a higher risk of preterm labor.
3. Cervical Issues: A short cervix or cervical incompetence can contribute to preterm labor.
4. Placental Problems: Issues with the placenta, similar as placental abruption or placenta previa, can lead to preterm birth.
5. Chronic Conditions: Conditions like diabetes and high blood pressure can increase the risk of preterm labor.
6. Stress and Lifestyle Factors: High levels of stress, smoking, drug use, and inadequate prenatal care can all contribute to preterm labor.

Risk Factors for Preterm Labor:

Several threat factors can increase the liability of preterm labor:

- Previous Preterm Birth: If a woman has previously given birth prematurely, her risk is higher.
- Multiple Pregnancies: As mentioned earlier, carrying twins, triplets, or more increases the risk.
- Infections: Infections of the amniotic fluid or lower genital tract can lead to preterm labor.
- Short Cervix: A cervix shorter than normal may not be able to support a full-term pregnancy.
- Age: Women under 18 and over 35 are at an advanced threat
- Race/Ethnicity: Some racial and ethnic groups have higher rates of preterm birth.

Symptoms of Preterm Labor:

Recognizing the signs of preterm labor is crucial. Common symptoms include:

- Regular Contractions: Contractions that occur at regular intervals, increasing in strength and frequency.
- Lower Back Pain: Persistent or intermittent back pain.
- Abdominal Cramps: Pain in the lower abdomen.
- Changes in Vaginal Discharge: An increase in vaginal discharge, especially if it's watery, mucus-like, or bloody.
- Pelvic Pressure: A feeling of pressure in the pelvis.
- Fluid Leakage: The leaking of amniotic fluid.

Management of Preterm Labor:

When preterm labor is suspected, it is essential to seek medical attention immediately. Healthcare providers will use various methods to assess the situation and determine the best course of action. These may include:

- Physical Examination: To check for signs of cervical dilation and contractions.
- Ultrasound: To measure cervical length and evaluate the baby's position.
- Fetal Monitoring: To assess the baby's well-being and contractions.
- Amniocentesis: To check for infection or lung maturity if birth is imminent.

Management options can include:

- Tocolytic Medications: These drugs can help delay labor temporarily by relaxing the uterine muscles.
- Corticosteroids: If preterm birth is imminent, corticosteroids can be given to help the baby's lungs develop faster.
- Bed Rest: In some cases, bed rest may be recommended to reduce the risk of further contractions.

- Cervical Cerclage: A surgical procedure to sew the cervix closed if it's deemed too short or weak.
- Hospitalization: In severe cases, the expectant mother may need to stay in the hospital for close monitoring.

Preventing preterm labor is not always possible, but good prenatal care, a healthy lifestyle, and early intervention when symptoms are noticed can help reduce the risk. Regular prenatal check-ups and open communication with healthcare providers are vital during pregnancy to address any potential issues promptly.

preterm labor is a complex and concerning issue in pregnancy. It can lead to adverse outcomes for both the baby and the mother. Recognizing risk factors, understanding symptoms, and seeking prompt medical attention are crucial steps in managing preterm labor and improving the chances of a healthy outcome for the baby.

8. HIGH BLOOD SUGAR LEVELS

Gestational Diabetes Risks & Management

High blood sugar levels during pregnancy can be a cause for concern and are typically referred to as gestational diabetes mellitus (GDM). This condition occurs when the body cannot produce enough insulin to meet the increased needs during pregnancy. Here, we'll discuss the causes, symptoms, risks, and management of high blood sugar levels in pregnancy.

Causes:

1. Hormonal Changes: During pregnancy, the placenta produces hormones that can interfere with the body's insulin function, leading to insulin resistance.

2. Genetics: A family history of diabetes or a history of GDM in a previous pregnancy can increase the risk of developing high blood sugar during pregnancy.

Symptoms:

Gestational diabetes often doesn't present noticeable symptoms. Sometimes, women may experience symptoms similar to those of diabetes, such as increased thirst, frequent urination, and fatigue.

Risks:

High blood sugar levels during pregnancy can have significant consequences for both the mother and the baby.

1. Maternal Risks:
   - Increased threat of developing type 2 diabetes later in life.
   - Preeclampsia, a situation characterized by high blood pressure and harm to other organs.
   - A need for a cesarean section due to complications during delivery.
2. Fetal Risks:
   - Macrosomia (large birth weight), which can result to birth injuries.
   - Hypoglycemia(low blood sugar) in the newborn after birth.
   - Respiratory distress syndrome in the baby.
   - Increased risk of the child developing obesity and type 2 diabetes later in life.

Management:

The goal in managing high blood sugar levels during pregnancy is to keep blood glucose within a target range to reduce risks. There are some crucial aspects of managing gravid diabetes

1. Diet and Nutrition: A registered dietitian can help create a customized meal plan that controls blood sugar levels.
2. Regular Monitoring: Regularly checking blood glucose levels is essential. This may involve self-monitoring at home or more frequent visits to a healthcare provider.
3. Physical Activity: Incorporating safe and regular physical activity into the daily routine can help control blood sugar.
4. Insulin or Medications: In some cases, insulin or other medications may be prescribed to control blood sugar levels.
5. Prenatal Care: Attending all prenatal appointments and working closely with

healthcare providers is crucial to monitor and manage gestational diabetes effectively.

6. Fetal Monitoring: Physicians may recommend additional monitoring, such as non-stress tests or ultrasounds, to ensure the well-being of the baby.

7. Postpartum Follow-Up: After delivery, it's essential to continue monitoring blood sugar levels as women with GDM have a higher risk of developing type 2 diabetes in the future.

High blood sugar levels during pregnancy, or gestational diabetes, is a condition that requires careful management to reduce the associated risks for both the mother and the baby. With proper care, many women with gestational diabetes can have healthy pregnancies and deliver healthy babies. If you suspect or have been diagnosed with gestational diabetes, it's essential to work closely with your healthcare team to develop a comprehensive management plan.

9. DEPRESSION AND ANXIETY

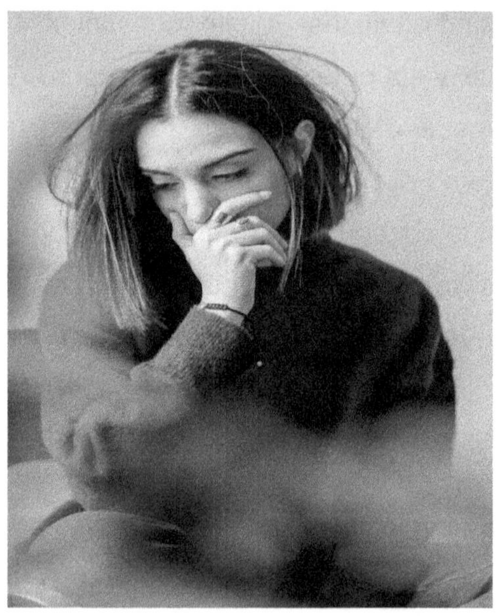

Depression and anxiety during pregnancy, often referred to as perinatal depression and anxiety, are significant mental health issues that can affect pregnant individuals. These conditions can have serious implications for both the expectant mother and the developing fetus. Understanding the causes, symptoms, risks, and treatment options is crucial for addressing this issue.

Causes of Depression and Anxiety in Pregnancy:

1. Hormonal Changes: Pregnancy leads to significant hormonal fluctuations, which can affect mood and emotions. Changes in estrogen and progesterone levels can impact neurotransmitters in the brain, contributing to mood disorders.

2. Emotional Stress: The anticipation of becoming a parent, financial worries, relationship concerns, and fear of childbirth are common stressors during pregnancy that can trigger anxiety and depression.

3. Previous Mental Health History: Individuals with a history of depression or anxiety are at a higher risk of experiencing these conditions during pregnancy. Previous trauma or unresolved emotional problems can also contribute.

4. Social and Environmental Factors: Lack of support, a stressful home environment, or inadequate access to healthcare can exacerbate perinatal mental health issues.

Symptoms of Depression and Anxiety in Pregnancy:

1. Persistent Sadness or Irritability: Feeling down most of the time, or frequent mood swings.
2. Changes in Sleep Patterns: Insomnia or excessive sleep can be symptoms of these conditions.
3. Appetite Changes: Notable changes in appetite or weight can occur.
4. Lack of Interest: A diminished interest in activities one previously enjoyed.
5. Fatigue: Feeling excessively tired or lacking energy.
6. Physical Symptoms: Headaches, muscle aches, and other physical complaints.
7. Worry and Anxiety: Excessive worry, fear, and anxiety about pregnancy, childbirth, or parenting.
8. Difficulty Concentrating: Finding it hard to focus or to make decisions.

Risks and Impact on Pregnancy:

1. Preterm Birth: Untreated depression and anxiety can increase the risk of preterm birth and low birth weight.
2. Developmental Issues: A baby's cognitive and emotional development may be affected if the mother is experiencing severe depression or anxiety.

Treatment Options:

1. Therapy: Cognitive-behavioral therapy (CBT) and interpersonal therapy are effective in treating perinatal depression and anxiety.
2. Medication: In some cases, medication may be prescribed under the supervision of a healthcare provider.
3. Support Groups: Joining support groups can help individuals connect with others facing similar challenges.

4. Self-Care: Engaging in self-care practices such as regular exercise, Reading good books, a balanced diet, and mindfulness can be beneficial.
5. Psychoeducation: Learning about perinatal mental health issues and their management is crucial.

Seeking Help:

If you or someone you know is experiencing depression or anxiety during pregnancy, it's important to seek help. Speak to a healthcare provider or internal health professional. Early intervention and support can make a significant difference in the well-being of both the expectant mother and the baby. Remember that you're not alone, and there are resources available to provide the necessary support during this challenging time.

10. SEVERE ITCHING

Severe itching during pregnancy can be a distressing symptom, and it often requires medical attention. It is essential to understand that intense itching can be a sign of an underlying medical condition known as intrahepatic cholestasis of pregnancy (ICP) or obstetric cholestasis. Here's an extensive overview of severe itching during pregnancy:

1. Understanding Severe Itching in Pregnancy:
    - Severe itching, especially on the palms and soles, is a common symptom of ICP.
    - ICP is a liver disorder that occurs during pregnancy and can lead to complications for both the mother and the baby.
2. Symptoms of ICP:

- The primary symptom is intense
    itching, which can range from mildly
    annoying to severely distressing.
  - Itching often worsens at night and
    can be so intense that it disrupts
    sleep.
  - Other signs may include dark urine,
    pale stools, and yellowing of the skin
    and eyes.
3. Causes of ICP:
  - The exact cause of ICP is not fully
    understood, but it's thought to be
    related to hormonal changes during
    pregnancy.
  - Genetics can also play a role; if a
    family member has had ICP during
    pregnancy, you may be at higher
    risk.
4. Complications:
  - ICP can increase the risk of preterm
    birth, fetal distress, and stillbirth.
  - There is also an increased risk of
    meconium staining (the baby
    passing stool before birth), which

can lead to respiratory problems in the newborn.

5. Diagnosis:
   - Diagnosis is typically based on symptoms, blood tests to check liver function, and measuring bile acid levels in the blood.
   - Other conditions that can cause itching, such as allergies and skin conditions, should be ruled out.

6. Treatment and Management:
   - The primary goal is to relieve symptoms and avert complications.
   - Medications such as ursodeoxycholic acid (UDCA) may be prescribed to reduce bile acids in the blood.
   - Regular monitoring of the baby's well-being through non-stress tests and ultrasound is essential.
   - Inducing labor may be considered if the risks to the baby become significant.

7. Self-Care:
    - While medical treatment is necessary, you can also try to alleviate itching by keeping your skin well-moisturized, taking cool baths, and avoiding hot water.
    - Avoid scratching to prevent skin damage and infections.
8. Follow-Up:
    - After pregnancy, symptoms of ICP usually resolve. However, you may be at a slightly higher risk for liver problems in the future.
9. Prevention:
    - If you have a family history of ICP, discuss it with your healthcare provider before getting pregnant.
    - Early detection and management are crucial for a healthy pregnancy outcome.

10. Consult a Healthcare Professional:

- If you experience severe itching during pregnancy, it's essential to consult with your healthcare provider promptly. They can perform the necessary tests and recommend appropriate treatment to ensure the well-being of both you and your baby.

Remember that while severe itching can be distressing during pregnancy, early diagnosis and medical management can significantly improve outcomes for both the mother and the baby. Always seek guidance from a healthcare professional for proper evaluation and care.

11. LEAKAGE OF AMNIOTIC FLUID

Amniotic Fluid Leakage Risk

Leakage of amniotic fluid during pregnancy, known as "premature rupture of membranes" (PROM), is a serious medical concern. Amniotic fluid plays a crucial role in protecting the developing fetus and facilitating its growth, making the loss of this fluid a potentially risky situation. Here's an extensive overview of this topic:

1. Amniotic Fluid Composition and Function:
   - Amniotic fluid is a clear, slightly yellowish liquid that surrounds the fetus within the amniotic sac.
   - It consists of water, electrolytes, proteins, and fetal waste products and is produced by both the mother and the developing fetus.

- Amniotic fluid serves multiple
  essential functions, including
  cushioning the fetus, maintaining a
  stable temperature, preventing the
  umbilical cord from being
  compressed, and allowing the fetus
  to move and develop properly.
2. Causes of Amniotic Fluid Leakage:
   - Premature rupture of membranes
     (PROM) can occur for several
     reasons, including infections,
     trauma, or weakening of the
     amniotic sac.
   - In some cases, it may be caused by
     factors such as smoking, drug use,
     or certain medical conditions.
3. Diagnosing Amniotic Fluid Leakage:
   - The primary symptom of PROM is
     the leakage of amniotic fluid, which
     can be a slow, continuous trickle or a
     sudden gush.
   - Diagnosis is often confirmed through
     physical examination and testing,

including pH testing of the fluid to differentiate it from urine.

4. Risks and Complications:
   - PROM can increase the risk of infections, as the protective barrier against bacteria is compromised.
   - It can lead to premature birth, which may result in neonatal complications due to underdeveloped organs and systems.

5. Management and Treatment:
   - Treatment options depend on the gestational age, severity, and potential complications. In some cases, labor may be induced or a cesarean section performed.
   - Antibiotics are frequently administered to lower the risk of infection.

6. Expectant Management:
   - If PROM occurs close to full-term (after 37 weeks) and there are no signs of infection or other complications, doctors may choose

expectant management, allowing
labor to begin naturally.

7. Complications for the Mother:

    o Prolonged PROM can lead to an
      increased risk of chorioamnionitis,
      an infection of the fetal membranes,
      which may necessitate antibiotics
      and early delivery.

8. Complications for the Fetus:

    o The longer the time between PROM
      and delivery, the greater the risk of
      fetal complications, including
      respiratory distress syndrome (RDS)
      and intraventricular hemorrhage
      (IVH).

9. Prevention and Self-Care:

    o Staying healthy during pregnancy
      through proper prenatal care,
      avoiding risky behaviors, and
      promptly addressing any signs of
      infection can reduce the risk of
      PROM.

10. Conclusion:

- Premature rupture of membranes (PROM) is a critical issue during pregnancy. It requires close monitoring and medical attention to ensure the safety and well-being of both the mother and the developing fetus. Early diagnosis and appropriate management are key to minimizing potential risks and complications associated with amniotic fluid leakage. Pregnant women should always consult with their healthcare providers if they suspect they may have experienced PROM.

12. HIGH BLOOD PRESSURE

High blood pressure during pregnancy, also known as gestational hypertension or pre-existing hypertension in pregnancy, is a serious medical condition that can have significant implications for both the mother and the baby. In this response, I will provide an extensive overview of high blood pressure in pregnancy, covering its types, causes, symptoms, risk factors, complications, diagnosis, and management.

Types of High Blood Pressure in Pregnancy:

1. Gestational Hypertension: This type of high blood pressure develops for the first time during pregnancy and usually goes away after childbirth. It commonly happens after the 20th week of pregnancy.
2. Chronic Hypertension: Some women may have hypertension before they become pregnant, and this condition continues

during pregnancy. Chronic hypertension can increase the risk of complications.

3. Preeclampsia: Preeclampsia is a severe condition that can develop after the 20th week of pregnancy and is characterized by high blood pressure along with signs of organ damage, often involving the liver and kidneys.

4. Preeclampsia with Severe Features: This is a more severe form of preeclampsia, with additional complications like severe hypertension, blood clotting problems, and impaired liver and kidney function.

Causes of High Blood Pressure in Pregnancy:

The exact causes of high blood pressure during pregnancy are not always clear, but several factors may contribute, including:

- Genetics: A family history of high blood pressure can elevate the threat.

- Obesity: Being overweight or obese before pregnancy can rise the risk.
- Age: Women who are younger than 20 or older than 40 are at a higher threat.
- Multiple Pregnancies: Women carrying twins or more are at a higher risk.
- Pre-existing Conditions: Chronic hypertension, diabetes, and kidney disease can increase the likelihood of high blood pressure during pregnancy.

Symptoms:

High blood pressure in pregnancy can often be asymptomatic, but in some cases, it may lead to symptoms such as severe headaches, blurred vision, abdominal pain, swelling in the face and hands, and shortness of breath. These symptoms can be indicative of more severe conditions like preeclampsia.

Risk Factors:

Various risk factors can increase the likelihood of developing high blood pressure during pregnancy, including:

- First pregnancy
- Record of increased blood pressure in last pregnancies
- Family history of hypertension
- Obesity
- Multiple pregnancies (twins or more)
- Pre-existing medical illnesses such as diabetes or kidney disease

Complications:

High blood pressure in pregnancy can lead to a range of complications, both for the mother and the baby. Some of these complications include:

- Preeclampsia: Severe hypertension can lead to preeclampsia, which can result in organ damage and affect multiple systems in the body.
- Placental Abruption: High blood pressure can increase the risk of the placenta separating from the uterine wall before delivery, which can be life-threatening for both the mother and the baby.
- Preterm Birth: High blood pressure may lead to the need for early delivery, increasing the risk of premature birth and associated complications.
- Intrauterine Growth Restriction (IUGR): Insufficient blood flow due to hypertension can restrict the baby's growth.
- Stillbirth: Severe hypertension can increase the risk of stillbirth.

Diagnosis:

Diagnosis typically involves regular blood pressure monitoring during prenatal check-ups. Urine tests and blood tests are also performed to check for proteinuria and organ damage. Ultrasound may be used to monitor the baby's growth and well-being.

Management:

Managing high blood pressure in pregnancy involves a combination of lifestyle changes, medication, and close medical monitoring. Treatment may include:

- Lifestyle modifications: Maintaining a healthy diet, regular exercise practice , and proper weight management.
- Medications: Blood pressure medications may be prescribed if necessary.
- Close monitoring: Regular prenatal check-ups to track blood pressure and assess the baby's well-being.
- Hospitalization: In severe cases, hospitalization is advised.

High blood pressure during pregnancy is a complex condition that requires careful monitoring and management to minimize risks to both the mother and the baby. Regular prenatal care, lifestyle adjustments, and medical interventions are essential to ensure a healthy pregnancy and delivery. It's important for expectant mothers to work closely with their healthcare providers to manage high blood pressure effectively during this critical time.

13. UNEXPECTED OR EXCESSIVE WEIGHT GAIN:

Unexpected weight gain during pregnancy can be a cause for concern, as it may have implications for both the mother's and baby's health. While some degree of weight gain is a natural and necessary part of pregnancy, unexpected or excessive weight gain can lead to various complications.

1. Normal Weight Gain in Pregnancy: On average, a healthy woman with a normal pre-pregnancy BMI (Body Mass Index) is expected to gain between 25 to 35 pounds during pregnancy. This weight gain is distributed in the following order.
   - 7-8 pounds for the baby.
   - 1-2 pounds for the placenta.
   - 2-3 pounds for the amniotic fluid.
   - 2-4 pounds for increased blood volume.
   - 4-6 pounds for breast enlargement.

- o   5-9 pounds for stored fat for energy.

Causes of Unexpected Weight Gain:

2. a. Excessive Caloric Intake: Consuming more calories than the body needs can lead to weight gain. Some pregnant women may indulge in unhealthy eating habits, such as overeating or consuming high-calorie, low-nutrient foods.

    b. Fluid Retention: Swelling, or edema, is common during pregnancy, particularly in the third trimester. This can result in temporary weight gain due to excess fluid retention.

    c. Gestational Diabetes: Developing gestational diabetes can lead to increased weight gain. It can affect how the body processes sugar and lead to excess fat storage.

d. Hormonal Changes: Pregnancy
hormones, like estrogen and progesterone,
can affect metabolism and, in some cases,
lead to weight gain.

Risks of Excessive Weight Gain:

3. a. Gestational Hypertension: Excessive
weight gain can increase the risk of
gestational hypertension (high blood
pressure during pregnancy), which can be
harmful to both the mother and the baby.
b. Gestational Diabetes: As mentioned
earlier, excessive weight gain can contribute
to the development of gestational diabetes.
c. Complications During Labor: Heavier
women may face difficulties during labor
and childbirth, which can necessitate
medical interventions.
d. Postpartum Weight Retention: Excess
weight gained during pregnancy can be

challenging to lose postpartum, increasing
the risk of long-term obesity.

Managing Weight Gain:

4. a. Healthy Eating: Pregnant women should
focus on a well-balanced diet, including
plenty of fruits, vegetables, whole grains,
lean proteins, and healthy fats.
b. Regular Exercise: Staying physically
active during pregnancy, under a healthcare
provider's guidance, can help manage
weight gain and improve overall health.
c. Monitoring: Regular check-ups with a
healthcare provider can help monitor weight
gain and address any concerns early on.
d. Consulting a Dietitian: If unexpected
weight gain is a concern, seeking guidance
from a registered dietitian or healthcare
professional is advisable.

while some degree of weight gain is expected and necessary during pregnancy, unexpected or excessive weight gain can have health implications. It is essential for pregnant women to maintain a healthy lifestyle, monitor their weight, and seek guidance from healthcare professionals to ensure a safe and healthy pregnancy for both themselves and their babies.

14. SEVERE BACK PAIN

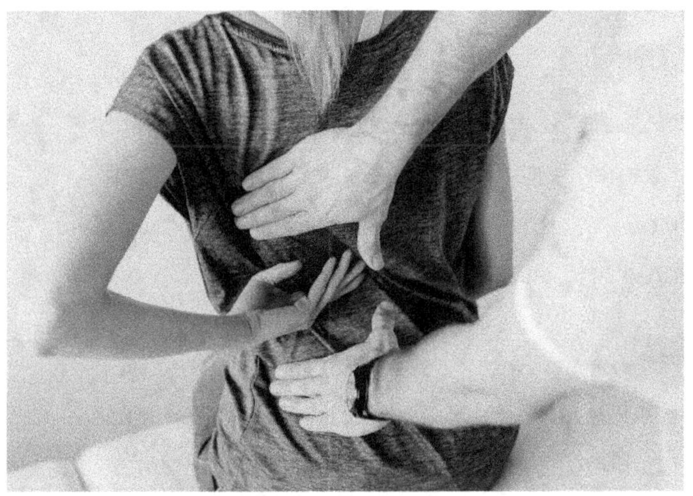

Severe back pain during pregnancy is a common complaint among expectant mothers. It can significantly impact a woman's quality of life during this crucial period. Several factors contribute to back pain during pregnancy, and there are various strategies to manage and alleviate the discomfort.

Causes of Severe Back Pain in Pregnancy:

a. Weight Gain: As a pregnancy progresses, a woman's weight increases. This puts extra pressure on the lower back, causing pain.

b. Hormonal Changes: Hormones like relaxin are released during pregnancy to help loosen the ligaments and prepare the body for childbirth. However, this can lead to instability in the pelvic area and back pain.

c. Posture Changes: As the belly grows, women tend to change their posture, which can strain the back muscles.

d. Center of Gravity: The shift in the body's center of gravity can place additional stress on the back.

Types of Back Pain in Pregnancy:

a. Lumbar Pain: This is the most common type and is felt in the lower back.

b. Pelvic Pain: This pain is typically felt in the front, in the pelvic region.

Managing Severe Back Pain:

a. Prenatal Exercises: Regular, gentle exercises that strengthen the back and core muscles can provide relief. Yoga and swimming are often recommended.

b. Proper Posture: Encouraging good posture and body mechanics can help reduce the strain on the back.

c. Supportive Maternity Wear: Wearing a maternity support belt can alleviate some of the pressure on the lower back.

d. Heat and Cold Therapy: Applying a heating pad or ice pack to the painful area can help reduce discomfort.

e. Massage and Physical Therapy: Professional help, like physical therapy or massage, can be beneficial in managing severe back pain.

f. Pain Medication: In some cases, a doctor may recommend safe pain relief options during pregnancy.

When to Seek Medical Attention:

If the back pain is severe, persistent, or accompanied by other symptoms like fever, chills, or numbness, it's essential to consult a healthcare provider. Severe back pain can be a sign of more serious conditions, such as sciatica, herniated discs, or preterm labor.

Preventing Back Pain During Pregnancy:

a. Maintain a Healthy Weight: Try to keep your weight gain within the recommended range.

b. Wear Supportive Shoes: Opt for comfortable, low-heeled shoes with good arch support.

c. Proper Lifting Techniques: Bend at the knees, not the waist, when picking up objects.

d. Stay Active: Regular, safe exercise throughout pregnancy can help prevent back pain.

Psychological Support: It's essential to recognize that severe back pain during pregnancy can be emotionally taxing. Seeking emotional support from family, friends, or a therapist can be valuable. Severe back pain during pregnancy is a challenging issue, but there are various strategies to manage and alleviate it. Every woman's experience is unique, so it's crucial to work with a healthcare provider to develop a personalized plan for pain management and ensure the safety and well-being of both the mother and the baby.

15. CHEST PAIN OR BREATHING DIFFICULTY

Chest pain and breathing difficulties during pregnancy can be concerning symptoms, and it's essential for pregnant individuals to be aware of their potential causes, when to seek medical attention, and how they can be managed. While I'll provide an extensive overview, it's crucial to remember that any chest pain or breathing difficulties during pregnancy should be discussed with a healthcare provider for proper evaluation and guidance.

Causes of Chest Pain and Breathing Difficulties in Pregnancy:

1. Physiological Changes: Pregnancy induces numerous physiological changes in the body, including an increase in blood volume, heart rate, and oxygen consumption. These

changes can lead to a feeling of breathlessness, especially in the later stages of pregnancy.

2. Heartburn: Many pregnant individuals experience heartburn, which can mimic chest pain. The pressure of the growing uterus on the stomach, hormonal changes, and relaxation of the esophageal sphincter can cause acid reflux, leading to chest discomfort.

3. Musculoskeletal Pain: As the uterus expands, it can put pressure on the diaphragm, causing chest pain or discomfort. Hormones like relaxin can also loosen ligaments, leading to musculoskeletal pain in the chest and ribcage.

4. Pulmonary Issues: Conditions such as asthma, bronchitis, or pneumonia can worsen during pregnancy, causing breathing difficulties. It's essential to manage these conditions with the guidance of a healthcare provider.

5. Preeclampsia: This is a potentially serious
    condition characterized by high blood
    pressure and damage to other organs.
    Symptoms can include chest pain,
    shortness of breath, and should be reported
    immediately to a healthcare provider.
6. Anxiety and Stress: Pregnancy can be a
    source of anxiety for many individuals.
    Stress and anxiety can manifest as chest
    pain and difficulty breathing. Techniques
    such as relaxation and stress management
    can help alleviate these symptoms.

When to Seek Medical Attention:

Any chest pain or severe breathing difficulties
during pregnancy should be taken seriously. Confer
a healthcare specialists   promptly if you experience
any of these:

- Sudden, severe chest pain.
- Chest pain accompanied by pain radiating
  to the jaw, left arm, or shoulder.

- Shortness of breath.
- Coughing up blood.
- Swelling in the legs, ankles, or feet.
- Rapid weight gain or severe headache, which can be indicative of preeclampsia.

Management and Prevention:

The management of chest pain and breathing difficulties during pregnancy will depend on the underlying cause. To alleviate some discomfort:

- Maintain good posture to help alleviate musculoskeletal pain.
- Eat smaller, more frequent meals to reduce heartburn.
- Avoid triggers for heartburn like spicy or fatty foods.
- Stay well-hydrated and perform light, regular exercise with the approval of your healthcare provider.

chest pain and breathing difficulties during pregnancy can arise from various causes. It's vital for pregnant individuals to stay in close communication with their healthcare providers, attend regular prenatal check-ups, and seek immediate medical attention if they experience severe or concerning symptoms to ensure a healthy and safe pregnancy

CHAPTER THREE

PREPARATION FOR DELIVERY

Preparing for labor and childbirth is a crucial aspect of a healthy and safe pregnancy. It involves a combination of physical, emotional, and practical preparations to ensure a smooth and successful delivery. While most labors progress without significant issues.

Preparations for Delivery:

1.Prenatal Education:

Enrolling in prenatal classes is an excellent way to prepare for delivery. These classes cover topics like stages of labor, pain management, breathing techniques, and postpartum care.

2.Choosing a Healthcare Provider:

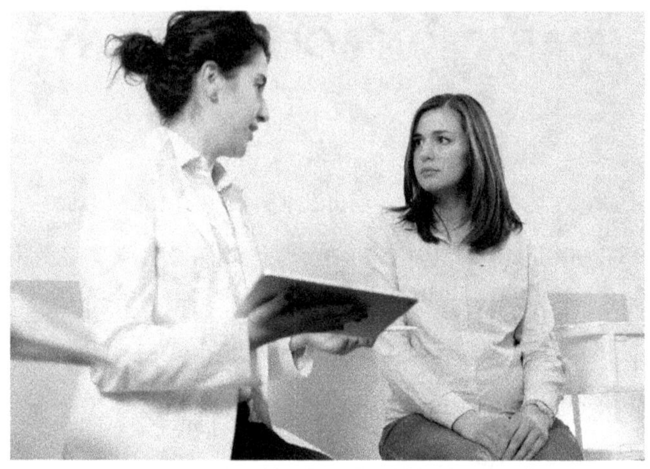

Select a trusted healthcare provider for your delivery. This could be an obstetrician, midwife, or a team of professionals. Ensure you're comfortable with their approach to labor and delivery.

3.Birth Plan:

Create a birth scheme outlining your choices for labor and delivery. This plan can include choices regarding pain management, birthing positions, and whether you want to labor in a hospital, birth center, or at home.

4.Packing Hospital Bag:

As your due date approaches, pack a bag with essentials for both you and the baby. This should include comfortable clothing, toiletries, snacks, and necessary documents.

5.Support System:

Discuss your birthing plans with your partner or chosen support person. Their emotional and physical support during labor can make a significant difference.

6.Nutrition and Exercise:

Preparing for delivery is an essential part of pregnancy, and maintaining a healthy diet and exercise regimen can contribute to a smoother pregnancy and childbirth. It's important to consult with a healthcare provider before making any significant changes to your diet or exercise routine during pregnancy, as individual needs can vary. However, here are some general guidelines for nutrition and exercise during pregnancy:

Nutrition:

- Balanced Diet: balanced diets are essential during pregnancy. Ensure you're getting a variety of nutrients, including carbohydrates, protein, healthy fats, vitamins, and minerals.
- Folate and Iron: These are critical nutrients for the development of your baby. Leaf vegetables , fortified cereals, and low fat meats are good sources.
- Calcium: Calcium is fundamental for the development of your baby's bones and teeth. Dairy products, leaf vegetables and fortified plant-based milk, are good sources.
- Fiber: Fiber can aid alleviate constipation, a common problem during pregnancy. Whole

grains, fruits, and vegetables are rich in fiber.

- Hydration: Staying hydrated is crucial. Take lots of water throughout the day to evade dehydration.

- Protein: Protein is vital for the development and growth of the baby. Good sources include lean meats, poultry, fish, eggs, and plant-based options like tofu and legumes.

- Healthy Snacking: Opt for nutritious snacks like fruits, yogurt, nuts, and whole-grain crackers to keep your energy levels stable.

- Avoid Processed Foods: Minimize the consumption of processed and sugary foods, as they can lead to excessive weight gain.

- Supplements: Prenatal vitamins, as recommended by your healthcare provider, can help fill in nutritional gaps.

Exercise:

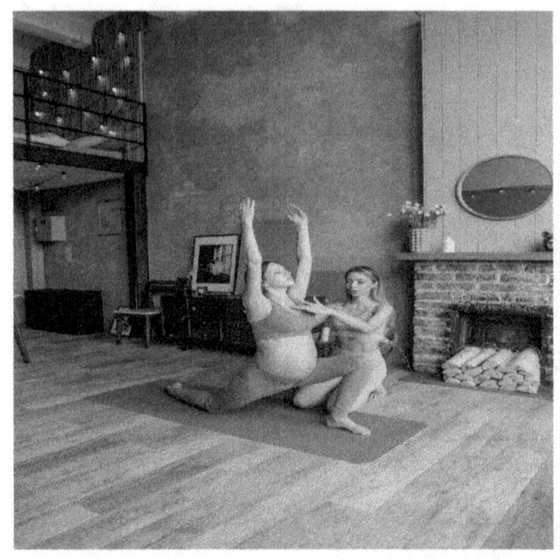

- Consult Your Healthcare Provider: Before beginning or continuing an exercise routine, consult your healthcare provider to ensure it's safe for you and your baby.
- Low-Impact Activities: Walking, swimming, and prenatal yoga are excellent low-impact exercises for maintaining fitness during pregnancy.

- Strength Training: Light strength training can help you build muscle, which can be

beneficial for carrying the extra weight of
pregnancy.

- Pelvic Floor Exercises: Kegel exercises can
  strengthen your pelvic floor muscles, which
  are crucial for labor and postpartum
  recovery.
- Listen to Your Body: Pay attention to your
  body's signals. If you feel fatigued, dizzy, or
  experience pain, stop and rest.
- Stay Cool: Exercise in a cool environment
  and wear loose, breathable clothing to
  prevent overheating.
- Avoid High-Risk Activities: Activities with a
  high risk of falling or injury, like contact
  sports, should be avoided.
- Posture: Focus on maintaining good posture
  to reduce strain on your back and pelvis.
- Relaxation: Incorporate relaxation
  techniques such as deep breathing or
  prenatal meditation to reduce stress and
  promote relaxation.

Remember every pregnancy varies, and what works for one individual may not work for another. It's essential to have open communication with your healthcare provider throughout your pregnancy journey to ensure you're making the best choices for your health and the health of your baby.

7.Pain Management:

Pain management during labor is a crucial aspect of childbirth, as it helps expectant mothers cope with the discomfort and pain associated with the birthing process. Various methods and techniques are available to assist women in managing pain during labor, ranging from non-pharmacological to pharmacological interventions. The choice of pain management should be individualized and based on the woman's preferences, medical history, and the progression of labor.

Non-Pharmacological Pain Management:

Breathing Techniques: Controlled breathing, such as the Lamaze method, can help women relax and focus during contractions.

Hydrotherapy: Soaking in a warm bath or using a shower can ease pain and help with relaxation.

Movement and Positioning: Changing positions frequently, such as walking or swaying, can alleviate discomfort.

Massage and Counterpressure: Gentle massages or counterpressure on the lower back can provide relief.

Visualization and Relaxation: Guided imagery and relaxation exercises can help women manage pain by diverting their focus.

Pharmacological Pain Management:

Epidural Anesthesia: An epidural is a common option, involving the injection of anesthetic medication into the epidural space to block pain in the lower half of the body. This provides substantial pain relief but may limit movement.

Spinal Block: Similar to an epidural, but provides quicker pain relief and is often used for cesarean sections.

IV Medications: Intravenous medications like opioids may be administered to lessen pain and help the woman relax. Nevertheless, they can have side impacts such as drowsiness.

Nitrous Oxide: Some hospitals offer nitrous oxide (laughing gas) to help with pain and anxiety during labor.

Combined Approaches:

Many women use a combination of non-pharmacological and pharmacological methods to manage pain. For example, they may start with relaxation techniques and then transition to epidural anesthesia if needed.

Supportive Care:

Emotional and physical support from a partner, doula, or midwife can play a significant role in pain management. Continuous support has been shown to reduce the need for medical interventions.

Individualized Approach:

Every woman's pain experience during labor is unique, and preferences for pain management can vary widely. Healthcare providers should work closely with expectant mothers to create a personalized pain management plan.

Informed Decision-Making:

It's essential for pregnant women to be well-informed about their pain management options and their potential benefits and risks. Discussing these options with healthcare providers, attending childbirth education classes, and having a birth plan can help in making informed decisions.

Monitoring Fetal Well-Being:

While managing pain is important, it's equally crucial to monitor the well-being of the baby throughout labor. Continuous fetal monitoring can help ensure the safety of both the mother and the child.

It's important to note that the choice of pain management during labor should be based on a woman's specific circumstances and desires. Healthcare providers will assess the progress of labor and provide guidance on the most appropriate methods for each individual case, taking into consideration factors such as the stage of labor, medical history, and the overall health of the mother and baby.

8. Understanding Stages of Labor and labor signs:

Labor is a complex process that can be divided into several stages, each with its own characteristics and milestones. The stages of labor typically include:

Stage 1: Early Labor(Latent Phase)

- Early labor can hold up for several hours or days.
- Contractions are usually mild and irregular during this stage.
- The cervix starts to efface and widen
- Women may experience backache, cramps, and other discomforts.

Active Labor:

- Contractions become stronger, more regular, and occur closer together.
- The cervix continues to dilate and efface.
- This stage typically lasts 6-12 hours for first-time mothers, and it can be shorter for subsequent pregnancies.
- Pain management options like epidurals may be considered.

Transition Phase:

- Transition is the most intense part of stage 1.
- Contractions are very strong and close together, lasting about 45-90 seconds.
- The cervix fully dilates (10 centimeters) during this phase.
- Women may feel overwhelmed and exhausted.

Stage 2: The Pushing Phase:

- This phase commences once the cervix is fully dilated.
- The mother starts actively pushing to move the baby through the birth canal.
- It can hold up from a few minutes to several hours.
- The baby's head becomes visible as it moves closer to delivery.

Birth of the Baby:

- o The baby's head appears, followed by the shoulders and the rest of the body.
- o This is the moment of birth.
- o The healthcare provider helps guide the baby if necessary.
- o The umbilical cord is usually cut.

Stage 3: Delivery of the Placenta:

- o After the baby is delivered, the placenta ought to be delivered.
- o The uterus goes on to contract to eject the placenta.
- o This stage typically takes a few minutes to 30 minutes.

Stage 4: Recovery:

- This stage is the immediate postpartum period.
- Healthcare providers monitor the mother for any bleeding or complications.
- Skin-to-skin contact with the baby may occur during this time.

Labor signs

Labor signs are important indicators that a woman's body is preparing for childbirth. These signs can vary in intensity and timing, but they generally follow a progression as the body gets ready for the delivery of a baby. Here, I'll provide an extensive overview of labor signs:

- Lightening: This is one of the early signs of labor, occurring a few weeks before delivery. The baby's head drops lower into the pelvis, relieving pressure on the diaphragm and making breathing easier.

This change in position can cause the pregnant woman to feel increased pressure in the pelvic area.

- Bloody Show: As the cervix begins to dilate and efface, a mucus plug that seals the cervix may be expelled. This mucus can be tinged with blood, creating a "bloody show." It's a sign that the cervix is preparing for labor.
- Contractions: Contractions are one of the most classic labor signs. They may start as Braxton-Hicks contractions, which are often irregular and painless, but they can become regular and more intense as true labor begins. True contractions become more frequent, longer, and stronger over time. Timing the contractions can help determine if it's true labor.
- Rupture of Membranes (Water Breaking): In some cases, the amniotic sac may rupture before contractions start. This is often depicted in movies with a dramatic gush of amniotic fluid, but in reality, it can be a slow

trickle. When this happens, it's essential to notify a healthcare provider.

- Back Pain: Many women experience back pain during labor, especially as the baby moves into the birth canal. This pain is usually more intense and frequent than typical back discomfort during pregnancy.
- Cervical Changes: As labor progresses, the cervix dilates and effaces. Cervical dilation refers to the opening of the cervix, while effacement indicates the thinning of the cervix. These changes are monitored by healthcare providers to track the progression of labor.
- Increased Discharge: Vaginal discharge can increase during labor. This is due to hormonal changes and the body's preparations for birth.
- Intestinal Changes: Some women may experience diarrhea or an upset stomach as their bodies prepare for labor. This is a natural response and is often referred to as the body "clearing out" before childbirth.

- Nesting Instinct: Some women experience a burst of energy and a strong desire to clean and organize their home shortly before labor begins. This is sometimes called the "nesting instinct" and can be a psychological sign of impending labor.
- Emotional Changes: Mood swings and heightened emotions are common as labor approaches. Anxiety, excitement, and anticipation are all normal feelings during this time.
- Engagement: Engagement refers to the baby's head moving down into the pelvis. It's a sign that the baby is getting into the proper position for birth. This can lead to increased pelvic pressure and the feeling of the baby "droppings or complications that may arise.
- Pelvic Pressure and Rectal Pressure: As the baby moves lower, women may feel increased pressure in the pelvic region and sometimes even rectal pressure. This can indicate that labor is advancing.

It's important to note that every woman's experience of labor is unique. Some may not experience all of these signs, and the order and intensity of signs can vary. If you believe you're experiencing signs of labor, it's crucial to contact your healthcare provider for guidance and support throughout the labor

9. Birth Environment:

- o Make choices about the birth environment, such as whether you want a home birth, a hospital, or a birthing center. Ensure you're comfortable with the setting.

10. Emotional Readiness:

- o Mentally prepare for the birthing experience. Acknowledge fears and uncertainties and discuss them with

your healthcare provider or a
counselor.

Remember that childbirth can be unpredictable, and it's essential to remain flexible and open to changes in your birth plan. Preparation helps, but ultimately, the safety and well-being of both you and your baby are the top priorities. Engage in open communication with your healthcare provider throughout the process to ensure a positive delivery experience.

CHAPTER FOUR

Postpartum Care

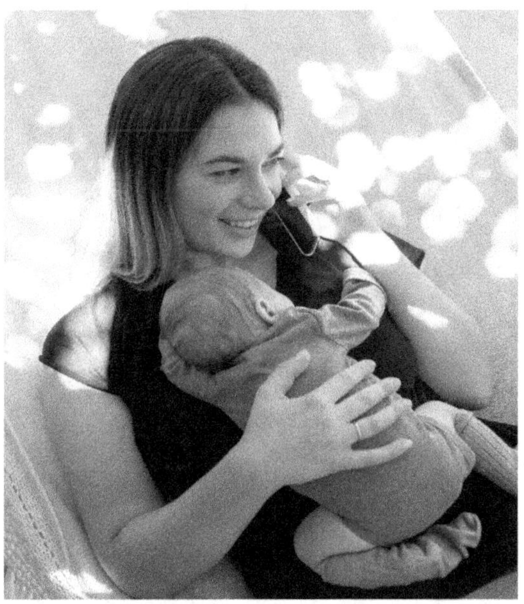

Postpartum care, also known as postnatal care, is a crucial aspect of maternal healthcare that focuses on the well-being of both the mother and her newborn in the period following childbirth. This care is essential to ensure the physical and emotional recovery of the mother and the healthy development of the baby. Here, we'll discuss postpartum care comprehensively, covering various aspects of this crucial phase.

1.Physical Recovery:

- **Monitoring**: Regular check-ups and assessments to track the mother's physical recovery, including uterine involution (the process of the uterus returning to its pre-pregnancy size), episiotomy or cesarean incision healing, and vital signs.
- **Pain Management**: Providing pain relief options for discomfort associated with childbirth, including medications or alternative therapies.Pain management after childbirth, especially during the postpartum period, is essential for the comfort and well-being of the

mother. Here are some common approaches to manage pain during postpartum care:

- Over-the-Counter Pain Medications: Non-prescription pain relievers like acetaminophen (Tylenol) or ibuprofen (Advil, Motrin) can help manage mild to moderate pain.
- Prescription Medications: For more severe pain, healthcare providers may prescribe stronger pain medications. Ensure you take these medications as directed by your healthcare experts.
- Epidural or Spinal Anesthesia: If you had an epidural or spinal block during labor, you might experience numbness that can provide pain relief during the early postpartum period.
- Local Anesthetics: Local anesthetics may be used for pain relief after episiotomy or perineal tears.

- Ice Packs: Applying ice packs to sore areas, such as the perineum or breasts, can help reduce pain and swelling.
- Warm Compresses: Warm compresses can be soothing and reduce discomfort, especially for engorged breasts or uterine cramps.
- Non-Pharmacological Methods: Techniques like deep breathing, relaxation exercises, and distraction can help manage pain and discomfort without medication.
- Rest: Adequate rest and sleep are essential for postpartum recovery and can alleviate fatigue-related discomfort.
- Hydration and Nutrition: Staying well-hydrated and eating balanced, nutritious meals can promote healing and overall well-being.
- Support: Emotional backing from relatives, close friends , or support groups can relieve the emotional

and psychological aspects of postpartum pain.

- Perineal Care: For mothers who have had vaginal births, perineal care is crucial. This includes keeping the area clean, applying ice packs to reduce swelling, and using pain relief medications as needed.
- Cesarean Section Care: Mothers who have had cesarean sections need extra care as they recover from major abdominal surgery. This includes monitoring the incision site and providing appropriate pain management.
- Nutrition: Recommending a balanced diet to support healing and milk production for breastfeeding mothers.

2. Emotional Well-being:

- Postpartum Depression Screening: Assessing the mother for signs of postpartum depression and providing appropriate interventions if needed.

- Supportive Counseling: Offering emotional support and counseling to help mothers cope with the emotional challenges of motherhood.
- Peer Support Groups: Encouraging participation in postpartum support groups to connect with other new mothers and share experiences.

3. Breastfeeding Support:

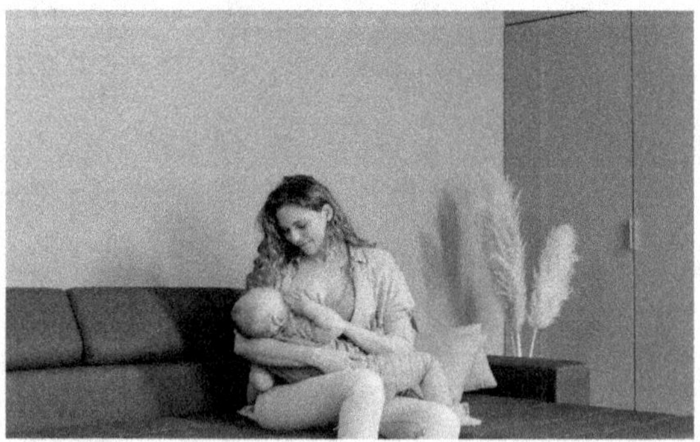

A. Lactation Consultation: Providing guidance on breastfeeding techniques, resolving breastfeeding challenges, and promoting the benefits of breastfeeding.Breastfeeding is a natural and essential way to nourish an infant, but it can come with a variety of challenges that new mothers may face. Understanding and addressing these challenges is crucial for the health and well-being of both the mother and the baby. Here are some common breastfeeding complications and how to manage them:

- Latch Issues: A proper latch is fundamental for successful breastfeeding. If the baby does not latch correctly, it can lead to sore nipples and difficulty in getting enough milk. To overcome this, mothers can seek assistance from a lactation consultant or a healthcare provider to ensure the baby is latching correctly.
- Sore Nipples: Sore or cracked nipples are common issues, especially in the early days of breastfeeding. To alleviate this discomfort, mothers can ensure a proper latch, use lanolin or other

nipple creams, and allow the nipples to air dry between feedings.

- o Low Milk Supply: Some mothers may worry about not producing enough milk to satisfy their baby's hunger. To increase milk supply, mothers should nurse on demand, stay well-hydrated, and consider pumping between feedings to stimulate more milk production.
- o Engorgement: Engorgement emerges when the breasts become excessively full, painful and overbearing . To relieve engorgement, mothers can nurse more frequently, apply warm compresses, or express a small amount of milk before nursing to soften the breast.
- o Plugged Ducts: A plugged milk duct can lead to discomfort and may even result in mastitis if not addressed. To clear a plugged duct, mothers can apply heat and massage to the

affected area, nurse on that side more frequently, and ensure the baby has a good latch.

- o Mastitis:This is an unbearable infection of the breast tissue, usually extremely painful. It may cause fever and flu-like symptoms. Mothers with mastitis should rest, continue breastfeeding, take prescribed antibiotics, and consult a healthcare provider for proper treatment.
- o Breastfeeding in Public: Some mothers may feel uncomfortable or anxious about breastfeeding in public. To overcome this challenge, it's essential to know your rights and become confident in breastfeeding discreetly. Nursing covers and clothing designed for breastfeeding can help.
- o Returning to Work: Balancing breastfeeding with a return to work can be challenging. Mothers can pump and store breast milk to

ensure their baby has a supply while they are away. Employers can help by providing proper facilities and break times for pumping.

- Breastfeeding Pain: Persistent pain during breastfeeding can be caused by a variety of factors, including thrush, tongue tie, or nipple vasospasms. Seeking help from a healthcare provider or a lactation consultant is essential for addressing the root cause.
- Weaning: Deciding when and how to wean your baby can be an emotional challenge. Mothers should choose a method that suits both their baby's needs and their comfort. Gradual weaning can be less traumatic for both mother and child.

B. Milk Supply Management: Assisting mothers in managing their milk supply, including addressing issues of low milk production or oversupply.

Milk management is crucial for new mothers who have recently given birth, as it ensures the well-being of both the mother and the baby. Here are some important tips for milk management:

- Breastfeeding: Breast milk is the best source of nutrition for newborns. Ensure that you breastfeed your baby regularly, ideally on demand, to establish a strong milk supply. Frequent feedings help stimulate milk production.
- Proper Latch: Ensure your newborn is latching rightly. A good latch ensures that your baby is getting enough milk and prevents nipple soreness.
- Hydration and Nutrition: Stay properly hydrated and retain a balanced diet. Proper nutrition is essential for milk production.

Consume foods rich in nutrients and calories, and consider consulting a lactation specialist for dietary advice.

- Rest and Relaxation: Get adequate rest and reduce stress as much as possible. Stress can negatively impact milk production. Take breaks and ask for help from family and friends when needed.
- Breast Pump: Consider using a breast pump to express and store extra milk. This can be useful for feeding when you're not available or if you have an oversupply of milk.
- Storage and Handling: If you're storing breast milk, do so in clean, sterile containers. Label them with dates and use the oldest milk first. Follow proper storage guidelines to maintain the milk's quality.
- Supplements and Medications: Consult your healthcare provider before taking any supplements or medications to increase milk supply.

They can recommend secure and effective options.

- Seek Support: Join support groups or consult a lactation consultant for guidance. Surround yourself with a support system that understands the challenges and can provide encouragement.
- Skin-to-Skin Contact: Practicing skin-to-skin contact with your newborn is very essential . This not only helps with bonding but also stimulates milk production.
- Pumping and Nursing Schedule: Establish a consistent schedule for nursing and pumping, but be flexible to accommodate your baby's needs. A routine can help maintain a steady milk supply.

Remember that every mother's milk production varies, and it's essential to focus on the well-being of both you and your baby. If you encounter challenges with milk management, consult with a healthcare professional or a lactation specialist for personalized guidance and support

4. Newborn Care:

- o Neonatal Care: Ensuring the newborn is healthy and thriving, including monitoring weight gain, feeding patterns, and developmental milestones.
- o Immunization Schedule: Advising parents on the recommended immunization schedule for the baby.
- o Educational Resources: Providing information on newborn care, including infant CPR, safe sleep practices, and colic management.

5. Contraception:

Discussing contraception options and family planning to help the mother make informed decisions about future pregnancies.Contraception in postpartum care is an important consideration for women who want to delay or avoid future pregnancies after giving birth. There are several options available:

- Barrier Methods: Barrier methods like condoms and diaphragms can be used immediately after childbirth and provide protection against pregnancy.
- Birth Control Pills: Some women can start birth control pills a few weeks after delivery, but it's essential to consult with a healthcare provider.
- Intrauterine Devices (IUDs): IUDs can be inserted shortly after childbirth, either immediately or at

the postpartum checkup. They offer long-term protection.

- o Contraceptive Implants: Hormonal implants like Nexplanon can be placed in the arm during the postpartum period.
- o Depo-Provera Injection: The contraceptive shot can be administered soon after childbirth, but it's important to consider the timing with your healthcare provider.
- o Breastfeeding: Exclusive breastfeeding can act as a natural contraceptive method, known as the Lactational Amenorrhea Method (LAM). However, it's not foolproof and requires strict adherence to specific criteria.
- o Tubal Ligation: If a woman is certain she doesn't want more children, tubal ligation (sterilization) can be performed, often during a cesarean section or postpartum.

6 .Physical Activity and Exercise:

Recommending postpartum exercises to help the mother regain strength and fitness safely. Physical activity and exercise play a crucial role in postpartum care, benefiting both the physical and mental well-being of new mothers. Here are some impacts of physical activities and exercises:

- o Recovery and Healing: After giving birth, the body goes through significant changes. Gentle, postpartum-specific exercises can help in the recovery process, reduce swelling, and improve circulation.
- o Strengthening Core Muscles: Pregnancy can weaken abdominal and pelvic floor muscles. Targeted exercises, such as Kegels, can help rebuild core strength, improve posture, and reduce back pain.

- Weight Management: Engaging in regular physical activity aids in shedding excess pregnancy weight and achieving a healthy body mass index. Combined with a balanced diet, it can help new mothers reach their pre-pregnancy weight.
- Stress Relief: The postpartum period can be emotionally taxing. Exercise triggers the release of endorphins, which can alleviate stress, anxiety, and postpartum depression.
- Energy Boost: Despite sleepless nights, exercising can provide an energy boost by improving cardiovascular health and increasing stamina.
- Social Support: Joining postnatal fitness classes or groups can offer social support, allowing new mothers to connect with others who are experiencing similar challenges.
- Improved Sleep: Regular physical activity can help regulate sleep

patterns, making it easier for new
mothers to get the rest they need.

- o Bonding with Baby: Some exercises, like yoga and baby-wearing workouts, allow mothers to bond with their infants while staying active.
- o Preventing Long-term Health Issues: Regular exercise can reduce the risk of long-term health issues such as cardiovascular disease, diabetes, and osteoporosis.

Key factors to note about postpartum exercises

- o Consultation with Healthcare Provider: It's essential for new mothers to consult their healthcare provider before starting any exercise routine, especially if they had a complicated pregnancy or delivery.

- Start Slowly and Progress Gradually:
  Begin with low-impact exercises and
  increase intensity over time. Pay
  attention to your body and don't
  propel yourself too hard initially.
- Balancing Rest and Activity:
  Adequate rest is crucial. New
  mothers should not overexert
  themselves, especially in the early
  postpartum weeks.

Postpartum exercises can help new mothers regain their strength and fitness after giving birth. It's important to consult with a healthcare professional before starting any exercise routine postpartum, as the timing and type of exercises can vary based on individual circumstances. Here are some examples of postpartum exercises:

1. Kegel exercises: These help strengthen the pelvic floor muscles, which can be weakened during pregnancy and childbirth.

2. Pelvic tilts: These help to strengthen the core and lower back muscles.

3. Gentle yoga: Prenatal and postnatal yoga classes can be beneficial for flexibility, relaxation, and toning muscles.

4. Walking: A low-impact exercise like walking can be a great way to start rebuilding stamina and maintaining a healthy weight.

5. Swimming: Swimming and water aerobics gives a low-impact, full-body workout.

6. Diaphragmatic breathing: Practicing deep breathing can help improve core strength and aid in relaxation.

7. Low-impact aerobics: Consider classes specifically designed for postpartum women to get back into cardiovascular shape.

8. Strength training: Using light weights or resistance bands can help tone and strengthen muscles.

9. Bodyweight exercises: Incorporate exercises like squats, lunges, and modified push-ups to target various muscle groups.

10. Postnatal fitness classes: Joining a postnatal fitness class, such as postnatal

Pilates or postnatal boot camp, can provide structured workouts designed for new mothers.

7. Family Planning:

Offering information and support for family planning, including discussions about birth control options and fertility awareness.

8. Postpartum Check-ups:

Scheduling follow-up visits to ensure that both the mother and baby are progressing well and addressing any concerns or complications that may arise.

9 .Support at Home:

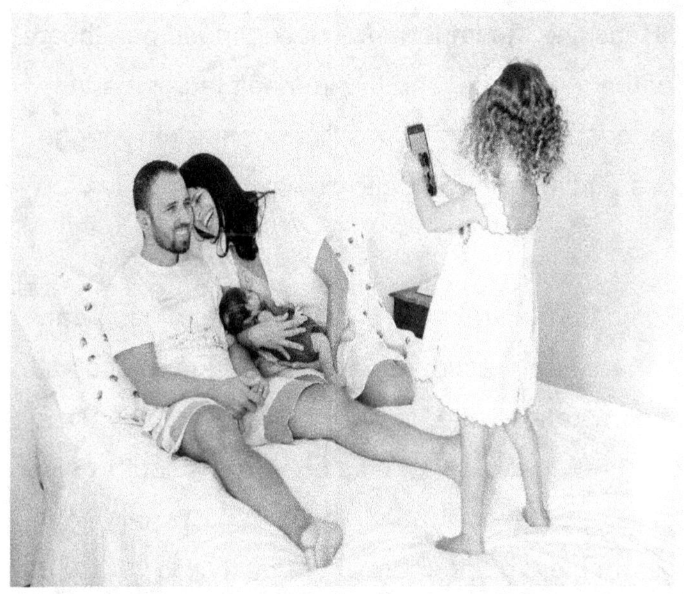

Encouraging a supportive and nurturing environment at home, including the involvement of partners and family members.

10 .Long-Term Health:

Discussing the importance of continued healthcare for the mother beyond the immediate postpartum period, addressing issues like postpartum weight loss and long-term health goals.

Postpartum care is not a one-size-fits-all approach. It should be personalized to the unique needs and circumstances of each mother and her baby. This comprehensive care helps ensure a smooth transition to motherhood, fosters emotional well-being, and promotes the health and development of the newborn. It is a critical component of maternal and child healthcare, contributing to the long-term health and happiness of the family.

CONCLUSION

Pregnancy is a remarkable journey in a woman's life, characterized by physical and emotional changes as a new life develops within her. Throughout this process, it is crucial to remain vigilant and aware of potential red flags that may indicate underlying health concerns for both the mother and the developing fetus. In this discussion, we have explored various pregnancy red flags, emphasizing their significance in ensuring a safe and healthy pregnancy.

First and foremost, it is important to recognize that pregnancy red flags should never be taken lightly. They serve as warning signs that demand immediate attention and medical evaluation. Whether it's spotting or bleeding, severe abdominal pain, or a sudden increase in blood pressure, these indicators can be early signs of complications that, if left unaddressed, may pose serious risks to the health of the mother and the unborn child.

The importance of regular prenatal care cannot be overstated. Prenatal visits are an essential component of a healthy pregnancy, as healthcare providers can monitor the progress of the pregnancy and address any red flags that may arise. It is vital for expectant mothers to adhere to their recommended prenatal care schedule, which typically involves frequent check-ups and various tests to identify potential issues early on.

Furthermore, communication is key. Mothers should maintain open and honest communication with their healthcare providers about any symptoms or concerns they may experience during pregnancy. Timely reporting of red flags is essential in ensuring swift and appropriate medical intervention, reducing the risks associated with complications.

In conclusion, recognizing and understanding the
Red flags in pregnancy is vital for the well-being of
both the pregnant individual and the developing
fetus. Pregnancy complications can arise from
various factors, including preexisting medical
conditions, infections, lifestyle choices, and genetic
factors. These complications can have a range of
effects, impacting maternal physical and emotional
health, as well as fetal and neonatal outcomes.

Early detection and prompt medical intervention are
key to managing these complications effectively.
Regular prenatal care, open communication with
healthcare providers, and adherence to
recommended treatment plans play a crucial role in
minimizing risks and optimizing outcomes.

Pregnancy is a unique journey, and while
complications can be concerning, with the right
care and support, many can be managed
successfully. Every pregnancy is different, and each
individual's experience may vary, but knowledge of

warning signs and proactive healthcare measures are essential in ensuring a safe and healthy pregnancy for both the expectant mother and the baby.Therefore, every expectant mother should prioritize her well-being and that of her child by staying informed, attending prenatal care appointments, and promptly reporting any red flags to her healthcare provider. By doing so, we can contribute to healthier pregnancies and ultimately, the well-being of the next generation.